SHOE YOGA FOR WEIGHT LOSS

Gay M. Fox

Table of Contents

CHAPTER1
Meaning of shoe yoga

Shoe Yoga is a novel and one-of-a-kind style of yoga in which participants perform a variety of yoga poses while wearing shoes. Due to its numerous advantages for the mind, body, and spirit, this relatively new style of yoga has gained popularity in recent years. Dissimilar to conventional yoga, which are ordinarily rehearsed shoeless, Shoe Yoga permits experts to wear shoes while performing yoga presents, which offer extra help and dependability to the feet and legs?

An experienced yoga instructor recognized the need for a more practical and comfortable form of yoga that could be practiced by people of all ages and fitness levels and came up with the idea for Shoe Yoga. Shoe Yoga's distinctive approach to yoga has earned it a significant following among yoga enthusiasts worldwide since its inception. Yoga is practiced with shoes that are made to be flexible, breathable, and comfortable. These shoes make it easy for practitioners to move around and do yoga poses.

CHAPTER2

Advantages of Shoe Yoga

One of the principal advantages of Shoe Yoga is that it assists with further developing equilibrium, adaptability, and strength. By wearing shoes while rehearsing yoga, professionals can keep up with legitimate arrangement and equilibrium, which lessens the gamble of injury and works on generally speaking execution. Additionally, Shoe Yoga is a great way to release body tension and stress, which can help you become more focused and clear-headed mentally. Shoe Yoga is a great way to improve your yoga practice and experience the many benefits of this ancient practice in a new and creative way, whether you are an experienced yogi or a beginner.

Shoe Yoga is a relatively new concept that combines modern footwear with the ancient practice of yoga. It is a holistic approach to footwear that focuses on the health and well-being of the feet, which has an impact on the body as a whole. The shoes are seen as an extension of the feet in Shoe Yoga, and the practice aims to create a supportive and comfortable environment in which the feet can flourish.

One of the fundamental standards of Shoe Yoga is the idea of "establishing." This is about the idea that the feet are the body's foundation and should always touch the ground. The shoes that are used in Shoe Yoga are made so that there is a natural connection between the feet and the ground, which makes it easier to stay in place and stay balanced. This may aid in injury prevention and enhance overall foot health.

Natural materials are used in Shoe Yoga, which is another important aspect. Shoes made of natural materials, like leather or cotton, are preferable to shoes made of synthetic materials because they let the feet breathe and can help prevent fungal infections and foot odor. Additionally, shoes that are made in accordance with the principles of Shoe Yoga frequently have a longer lifespan and are more durable than standard footwear.

In general, Shoe Yoga is an exceptional way to deal with footwear that spotlights on the wellbeing and prosperity of the feet. Shoe Yoga can support the principles of grounding and balance while also enhancing foot health and reducing the risk of injury by making use of natural materials and designing footwear that does so. Shoe yoga is a form of yoga that is practiced while wearing shoes. Whether you are an experienced yogi or just looking for a pair of shoes that are more comfortable and supportive, Shoe Yoga is definitely something you should look into. This may appear to conflict with traditional yoga practices, in which barefoot practice is common. However, in recent years, shoe yoga has gained popularity as a method for assisting people with foot injuries or problems to practice yoga without further harm. When practicing shoe yoga, participants put on shoes that are flexible and provide support while still allowing for proper alignment and balance.

The fact that shoe yoga permits people with foot issues to continue practicing yoga is one of its greatest advantages. Customary yoga stances can be challenging for those with conditions, for example, plantar fasciitis, bunions, or level feet. Shoe yoga can offer the vital help and padding expected to make these postures more available. Also, wearing shoes during yoga can give added foothold and soundness, which can be particularly useful for the people who battle with balance.

CHAPTER3

The potential benefits of shoe yoga

Shoe yoga has the potential to benefit all practitioners in addition to assisting those with foot issues. The additional cushioning and support can help prevent injury and alleviate joint pain. The shoes can also help keep the feet safe from fungal or bacterial infections that can spread from yoga studio floors. In general, shoe yoga can be a great choice for anyone who wants to improve their yoga practice and keep their feet safe from harm

Shoe yoga is a relatively new practice that enhances the practice's benefits by combining traditional yoga poses with shoes designed specifically for that purpose. Due to its capacity to assist individuals in achieving a wide range of health benefits, this distinctive form of exercise has been gaining popularity in recent years. One of the main benefits of shoe yoga is supporting weight reduction potential.

There are a number of ways shoe yoga can help you lose weight. First and foremost, the shoes utilized in this training are intended to offer additional help to the feet, which can assist with further developing equilibrium and security during yoga presents. This, in turn, may assist in increasing the workout's intensity, resulting in increased calorie burn and weight loss. Additionally, shoe yoga entails a wide variety of postures that work the core, legs, and arms. This full-body workout can help you lose weight over time by making your muscles stronger, speeding up your metabolism, and burning calories.

Additionally, stress and anxiety, which are frequently connected to overeating and weight gain, can be reduced through shoe yoga. It has been demonstrated that yoga helps lower cortisol levels, the stress-causing hormone, in the body. By diminishing feelings of anxiety, shoe yoga can assist with advancing good dieting propensities, decrease desires for unfortunate food varieties, and work on generally speaking mental prosperity. Better weight management and sustained weight loss over time may result from this, in turn.

In conclusion, shoe yoga is novel forms of exercise that can help people lose weight among other things. By further developing equilibrium, expanding force, reinforcing muscles, and decreasing pressure, shoe yoga can assist people with accomplishing their weight reduction objectives in a protected and powerful manner. With ordinary practice, shoe yoga can turn into a fundamental piece of a sound way of life, advancing in general physical and mental prosperity.

. Shoe yoga is a unique style of yoga in which participants practice yoga in their shoes. Due to its numerous advantages, including improved balance and posture, stress reduction, and increased flexibility, it is gaining popularity. Shoe yoga, on the other hand, can be quite challenging, particularly for beginners. We will go over some helpful hints in this article that will make it easier for you to practice shoe yoga.

Choosing the right shoes is the first step in doing shoe yoga. Shoes that are adaptable, supportive, and comfortable are essential. Your shoes ought to be light and spacious enough to permit your feet to move freely. Try not to wear shoes with high heels or thick soles, as they can influence your equilibrium and make it hard to accurately play out the stances. Additionally, to avoid slipping and falling during the practice, it is suggested to wear shoes with good grip.

The second piece of advice for shoe yoga is to start out slowly and build up the intensity of your practice over time. It's important to listen to your body and don't push yourself too far. Start with easy poses and work your way up to more difficult ones. If you are experiencing pain or discomfort, do not force yourself into a pose. If necessary, take breaks, and remember to breathe deeply throughout the exercise.

Finding a suitable space for your practice is the third piece of advice for doing shoe yoga. Choose a peaceful and quiet location where you can concentrate without being interrupted. In order to avoid accidents, make sure the floor is safe and clean. Cushioning and support for your feet can also be provided by using a towel or a yoga mat. You will notice improvements in your overall health and well-being if you practice shoe yoga at least three times per week.

In conclusion, shoe yoga is a great way to boost your mental and physical well-being. You can practice shoe yoga safely and effectively by following these guidelines. Remember to select the appropriate footwear, begin slowly, and select a suitable location for your practice. The numerous advantages of shoe yoga can be enjoyed with regular practice.

In yoga, the physical postures or positions of the body that are used to improve physical and mental health are called asana. One of a kind sort of yoga practice is Shoe Yoga, which includes performing asanas while wearing shoes. The goal of this type of yoga is to improve balance, coordination, and foot health in general. Asanas for Shoe Yoga can be drilled by people of any age and wellness levels, making it a flexible and open type of activity.

CHAPTER 4

Techniques and Types of shoe yoga

The Tree Pose, the Warrior Pose, and the Triangle Pose are among the most frequently practiced Asanas in Shoe Yoga. Standing in the Tree Pose, one must balance on one foot while the other foot rests on the inner thigh of the standing leg. The muscles in the lower leg and foot are strengthened and balance is improved as a result of this pose. Standing in the Warrior Pose, you lunge forward with one leg while extending the other leg behind you. This posture fortifies the legs and works on in general dependability. Standing in the Triangle Pose, one must extend one leg to the side and reach the opposite arm toward the foot of the extended leg. The foot and ankle muscles are strengthened and flexibility is improved in this pose.

It is essential to wear shoes that are appropriate for the style of yoga being practiced when performing Asanas for Shoe Yoga. For Asanas that demand balance and stability, shoes with a flat sole and adequate arch support are ideal. For Asanas that require flexibility and mobility, the best footwear is one with a flexible sole and ample cushioning. In addition, it is essential to make certain that the shoes fit correctly and are comfortable because shoes that don't fit right can cause pain or injury.

In general, Asanas for Shoe Yoga provide a one-of-a-kind and efficient method for enhancing foot health, balance, and coordination. By integrating these stances into a customary yoga practice, people can encounter the physical and mental advantages of yoga while likewise working on the wellbeing and strength of their feet. Anyone can practice Asanas for Shoe Yoga and reap the many benefits of this unique form of exercise if they use the right footwear and follow the correct technique.

Shoe Yoga is a novel and one-of-a-kind style of yoga that uses shoes as props to enhance the practice. Due to its numerous advantages, including improved flexibility, balance, and strength, this style of yoga is gaining popularity. Weight loss is one of Shoe Yoga's most important benefits. Shoe Yoga Asanas are a variety of postures that specifically target weight loss and, when practiced on a regular basis, can produce impressive outcomes.

The Chair Pose is one of the best Shoe Yoga Asanas for losing weight. To rehearse this asana, stand with your feet hip-width separated and your arms expanded above. As if you were sitting in a chair, flex your knees and lower your hips. Hold the posture for 30 seconds to a moment, and afterward discharge. The legs, hips, and core are all strengthened in the Chair Pose, which also aids in efficient calorie burning. One more successful Shoe Yoga Asana for weight reduction is the Fighter II Posture.

Stand with your feet wide apart and turn your right foot outward to perform this asana. Your arms should be extended out parallel to the ground as you bend your right knee. Repeat on the opposite side after holding the pose for 30 to 1 minute. In addition to effectively burning calories, the Warrior II Pose helps to tone the legs, hips, and thighs.

Additionally, the Tree Pose is a shoe yoga asana that helps people lose weight. To rehearse this asana, stand with your feet hip-width separated and put your right foot to your left side thigh. Repeat on the opposite side by bringing your hands together in front of your chest. Hold the pose for 30 to 1 minute. The legs and hips can be toned in the Tree Pose, which also helps improve balance and stability. When performed on a regular basis, this asana can assist in weight loss and effectively burn calories. Shoe yoga is a remarkable type of yoga that includes performing different asanas while wearing shoes. Yoga poses are made simpler for beginners by the stability and support provided by wearing shoes when practicing. In shoe yoga, you can do a variety of asanas, each of which has its own benefits. Here are a few nitty gritty guidelines for rehearsing every asana.

The Tadasana, or Mountain pose, is one of shoe yoga's most popular asanas. To perform this asana, stand straight with your toes pointing forward and your feet hip-width apart. Relax your shoulders and maintain a straight spine. Breathe deeply with your hands on your hips. Bring your arms up and over your head as you inhale. Reach upward with your fingers and arms. After a few deep breaths, let go of this pose.

The Warrior II pose is yet another fantastic asana for shoe yoga. To get started, stand in Tadasana and step your left foot back about three to four feet. Turn your left foot outwards, and your right foot somewhat inwards. Twist your right knee, keeping it straight over your lower leg. Stretch your arms out to the sides and up to shoulder height. Breathe deeply as you turn your head to look over your right hand. Repeat on the opposite side after remaining in this position for a few deep breaths.

Another excellent shoe yoga asana is the Chair pose. Start by standing in Tadasana and bending your knees so that you look like you're sitting on a chair. With your arms outstretched in front of you and your spine straight, After a few deep breaths, let go of this pose. The legs and core can be strengthened in the Chair pose, which also helps with balance and stability. You will notice a significant improvement in your overall health and wellbeing if you perform these asanas on a regular basis.

Any yoga practice, including shoe yoga, includes breathing exercises. Shoe yoga uses shoes as props to improve flexibility and balance. Shoe yoga can help increase relaxation, reduce stress, and improve lung capacity with the right breathing techniques.

Deep breathing is one of shoe yoga's most important breathing techniques. Breathing deeply through the nose and slowly through the mouth is known as deep breathing. This strategy assists with quieting the psyche and lessens pressure. Additionally, it contributes to an increase in the body's oxygen supply, which may increase lung capacity and overall health.

Ujjayi breathing is yet another important breathing technique in shoe yoga. Ujjayi breathing requires slightly constricting the back of the throat while inhaling and exhaling through the nose. This method can help you control your breathing and produce a soothing sound. Additionally, it can increase lung capacity and assist in increasing oxygen flow to the body.

In conclusion, the practice of yoga, including shoe yoga, relies heavily on breathing exercises. Shoe yoga can aid in stress reduction, relaxation, and increased lung capacity if done correctly. Probably the main breathing procedures in shoe yoga incorporate profound breathing and Ujjayi relaxing. You can reap all of the benefits of this ancient practice by incorporating these methods into your shoe yoga practice.

Breathing procedures are a fundamental piece of Shoe Yoga. These methods have numerous advantages that can assist individuals in improving their physical, mental, and emotional health. Stress reduction is one of the primary advantages of Shoe Yoga's breathing exercises. People can calm their minds and feel less stressed and anxious by focusing on deep, controlled breathing. People who struggle with depression or anxiety may particularly benefit from this.

Improved physical health is another advantage of Shoe Yoga's breathing techniques. Deep breathing can help increase oxygenation and lung capacity, both of which can lead to better health and more energy. In addition, people can reduce their risk of injury and pain by practicing proper breathing techniques and maintaining good posture.

At last, breathing methods in Shoe Yoga can assist people with working on their psychological and profound wellbeing. People can become more mindful and present in the now by concentrating on their breath. This can assist them with feeling more grounded and focused, which can prompt a more noteworthy feeling of by and large prosperity. Also, breathing exercises can help people become more aware of their thoughts and feelings, which can help them grow as people and become more aware of themselves.

Shoe Yoga is no exception to the rule when it comes to the importance of breathing techniques. Shoe Yoga practitioners use a variety of breathing techniques to maximize the practice's benefits. Deep breathing is one of Shoe Yoga's most common breathing exercises. Breathing deeply through the nose and slowly through the mouth is known as deep breathing. Increased oxygen intake, improved circulation, and decreased stress are all benefits of this method. During their practice, practitioners can also increase their sense of mindfulness and relaxation by concentrating on the breath.

One more breathing procedure utilized in Shoe Yoga is Ujjayi relaxing. Ujjayi breathing involves contracting the muscles in the throat while inhaling and exhaling through the nose. This method produces a soft hissing sound that aids in mind focus and deep breathing. Additionally, Ujjayi breathing enhances the flow of prana—the life force energy—throughout the body and increases lung capacity. Because it helps to calm the mind and keep the breath steady, this technique can be especially helpful in more difficult poses.

Finally, Nadi Shodhana, or alternate nostril breathing, is incorporated into Shoe Yoga. The thumb and ring finger are used to close one nostril at a time while simultaneously inhaling and exhaling through the other. Nadi Shodhana assists with adjusting the progression of prana all through the body and can be particularly valuable for diminishing pressure and tension. This method is useful for both yoga practice and everyday life because it also helps improve focus and concentration.

All in all, breathing procedures are a critical part of Shoe Yoga. Some of the techniques used in this practice to help practitioners achieve a deeper sense of relaxation, focus, and mindfulness include deep breathing, Ujjayi breathing, and Nadi Shodhana. Students can increase the physical and mental benefits of Shoe Yoga and achieve a greater sense of overall health and well-being by incorporating these methods into their practice.

Shoe Yoga is a type of yoga in which participants perform yoga poses while wearing shoes. It is a well-liked form of yoga that has recently gained a lot of popularity. The primary benefit of shoe yoga is that it enhances stability and balance during yoga practice. Utilizing breathing exercises is one of shoe yoga's most important elements. During yoga practice, these techniques help to calm the mind and improve focus.

It is essential to begin shoe yoga breathing exercises by sitting in a comfortable position with your shoes on. Take a few deep breaths in through your nose and out through your mouth to get started. Concentrate on expanding your chest and filling your lungs with air as you inhale. As you breathe out, center around delivering any pressure in your body and loosening up your psyche.

The Ujjayi breath is yet another effective shoe yoga breathing technique. To play out this procedure, begin by breathing in profoundly through the nose. As you breathe out, contract the rear of your throat somewhat to make a murmuring sound. You should be able to hear this sound, but others around you won't. During yoga practice, the Ujjayi breath helps to improve focus and energy.

Last but not least, it is essential to keep in mind to breathe slowly and deeply when practicing breathing exercises in shoe yoga. This helps the body get more oxygen and makes you feel more relaxed in general. During your shoe yoga practice, you can experience increased balance, stability, and relaxation by concentrating on your breath and incorporating these straightforward techniques.

Shoe yoga is a one-of-a-kind style of yoga in which participants practice yoga poses while donning shoes. People who want to improve their balance, flexibility, and overall health are starting to take this type of yoga more and more seriously. Breathing exercises are incorporated into shoe yoga, which is one of its most important features. Breathing methods are a fundamental piece of any yoga practice as they help to quiet the brain, diminish pressure, and further develop center.

The benefits of shoe yoga can be enhanced by including breathing exercises. Focusing on the breath and using it to direct movement is essential in shoe yoga. The Ujjayi breath is one of shoe yoga's most effective breathing exercises. With a slight constriction in the throat, this is a deep, slow breathing technique that involves inhaling through the nose and exhaling through the mouth. This way of breathing helps to calm the mind and increases the amount of oxygen that is taken in, which can make it easier to focus and last longer.

One more breathing strategy that can be consolidated in a shoe yoga practice is the Kapalbhati breath. This is a method of rapid breathing through the nose that uses forceful exhalation. Using kapalbhati breathing during a shoe yoga practice is a great way to energize the body and increase circulation. It is vital to make sure to begin slow and progressively increment the force of the breath as you become more OK with the strategy.

In conclusion, the unique benefits of shoe yoga can be enhanced by incorporating breathing exercises into the practice. By zeroing in on the breath and utilizing it to direct development, specialists can further develop equilibrium, adaptability, and generally speaking wellbeing. Whether you're using the Kapalbhati breath or the Ujjayi breath, it's important to start slowly and gradually increase the intensity of the breath as you get better at it. Shoe yoga and breathing exercises can improve mental and physical health with regular practice.

Yoga is a practice that can benefit anyone, no matter how old they are or how fit they are. You don't need any special equipment to incorporate yoga into your daily routine by creating a shoe yoga routine. You only need a pair of supportive shoes and the willingness to experiment.

CHAPTER5

Fundamental poses of shoe yoga routine

It is essential to begin a shoe yoga routine with a few fundamental poses that can be easily modified to meet your needs. For beginners, downward dog, warrior one, and tree pose are excellent options. You can move on to more challenging poses like the crow and headstand once you're comfortable with these ones. Listening to your body and only doing what makes you feel good are important.

One more significant part of making a shoe yoga routine is to zero in on your breath. During your practice, it can help you relax and stay focused by taking deep, mindful breaths. As you progress through each pose, try inhaling deeply through your nose and exhaling slowly through your mouth. You'll be able to stay present and connected to your body with this.

In general, developing a routine of shoe yoga is a great way to boost your strength, flexibility, and sense of well-being. You will begin to notice the benefits of yoga in your daily life with a little practice.

So on the off chance that you're searching for a method for integrating yoga into your daily practice, consider making a shoe yoga schedule today!

Making a shoe yoga routine is a great way to stretch, relax, and take care of your feet at the same time. Incorporating various asanas, or poses, that target various parts of the feet and legs, is one of the most important aspects of a shoe yoga routine. There are a wide range of asanas that can be remembered for a shoe yoga normal, each with their own advantages.

The downward dog is an excellent asana for a shoe yoga routine. In addition to strengthening the arms and shoulders, this pose helps to stretch the hamstrings and calves. Start on your hands and knees and lift your hips up toward the ceiling while keeping your hands and feet firmly planted on the ground to perform this pose. After a few deep breaths, let go of this pose.

The tree pose is yet another excellent asana for a shoe yoga routine. In addition to stretching the hips and legs, this pose aids in improving balance and stability. Standing with your feet hip-width apart, shift your weight onto one foot to perform this pose. Place the sole of your foot against the inside of your thigh as you bend the opposite knee. After a few breaths of balance here, release and switch sides.

Lastly, another great asana for a shoe yoga routine is warrior pose. In addition to stretching the hips and chest, this pose helps to strengthen the legs and core. Step forward with one foot and bend one knee while keeping the other foot on the ground to perform this pose. Hold this pose for a few breaths by raising your arms toward the ceiling, then switch sides and release. Integrating these and different asanas into your shoe yoga routine can assist you with feeling more loose and invigorated over the course of your day

Breathing methods are a fundamental part of an effective shoe yoga schedule. While also expanding your lung capacity, proper breathing techniques can help you relax and concentrate on the movements. Perhaps of the most well-known breathing procedure utilized in shoe yoga is called ujjayi breathing, which includes breathing in and breathing out through the nose while marginally tightening the rear of the throat. This procedure can assist you with keeping on track and quiet during your training.

Alternate nostril breathing is another breathing strategy used in shoe yoga. This includes utilizing your fingers to impede one nostril while breathing in through the other, then, at that point, exchanging and breathing out through the contrary nostril. The body and mind can be brought into harmony by this method, which can help regulate the flow of air between the nostrils. It's especially helpful when you're stressed or anxious.

Last but not least, you can incorporate deep breathing into your shoe yoga practice. This entails inhaling deeply through the nose and slowly exhaling through the mouth. It will be easier for you to concentrate on your movements and get the most out of your shoe yoga practice if you use this method to help you relax and let go of tension throughout your body. You can increase your sense of mindfulness and improve your overall well-being by incorporating these breathing exercises into your shoe yoga practice.

THE END